WHAT'S ZAPPING YOUR ENERGY?

5 health mistakes that are making you tired – and how to fix them

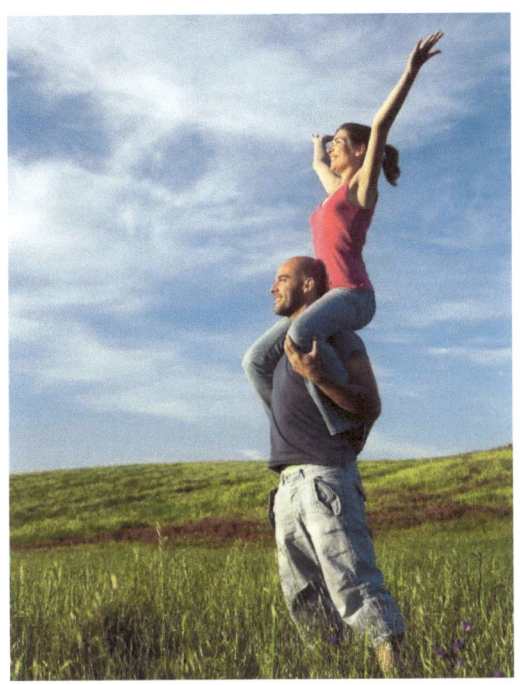

Image credit: 123RF Stock Photo

Dr. Michael Rahman, BSc, ND

Doctor of Naturopathic Medicine

Disclaimer

The content of this booklet is presented in summary form, is general in nature, and is provided for informational purposes only; it is not intended nor recommended as a substitute for professional medical advice. You should not use the content of this booklet for diagnosing a health problem or disease. Always seek the advice of your physician or other qualified health provider regarding any medical condition or treatment. Nothing contained in this booklet is intended to be for medical diagnosis or treatment. Never disregard medical advice or delay in seeking it because of something you have read in this booklet.

Acknowledgements

I would like to thank all those who have helped in making this booklet available for your education: my team at Pinewood Natural Health Centre, my office guru extraordinaire Cheryl Watson for coordination and David Ensuncho for his creative genius and ongoing support; lastly to Denise, editor and wordsmith, for helping make me sound less "doctor-ish." I'd like to extend a special acknowledgement to all the patients and families that have shared and taught me as much as I have taught them.

Toronto, 2014

Introduction
What makes us tired?

Chances are if you ask any adult the last time they woke feeling well rested, they won't be able to tell you. Most of us think this is because we don't sleep enough. After all, sleep sometimes takes a backseat to the demands of family, work, and home. But feeling well-rested is about more than just how much sleep we get. It is about our overall health: our diet, our hormones and our emotional health.

When we don't feel well-rested, it impacts every aspect of our health and well-being. It can exacerbate existing medical conditions, increase anxiety or depression, and lead to general irritability. In a nutshell, we feel zapped of energy.

If you've picked up this book, chances are that you feel tired – and you want to change that. This book is a great first step toward better health. Building your knowledge about the body and its systems – and how they all work together to contribute to your overall health – can be a very powerful and inspiring path.

This book is intended as a guide to help you isolate the factors in your life that might be making you tired, while providing practical suggestions for improving your health in each of these areas. As a naturopathic doctor at Pinewood Natural Health Centre, every day I see what happens when patients start taking control of their health and well-being. The results are awe-inspiring and truly remarkable. At Pinewood we help people just like you find natural ways to overcome their loss of energy and emerge with a new zest for life.

The purpose of this book is to empower you to make positive changes in your life that will lead to a lasting transformation that leaves you feeling happy, alert, and energized.

Dr. Michael Rahman, Toronto, 2014

Table of Contents

Mistake #1: Your Diet Needs an Overhaul
The problem: Your diet isn't properly balanced

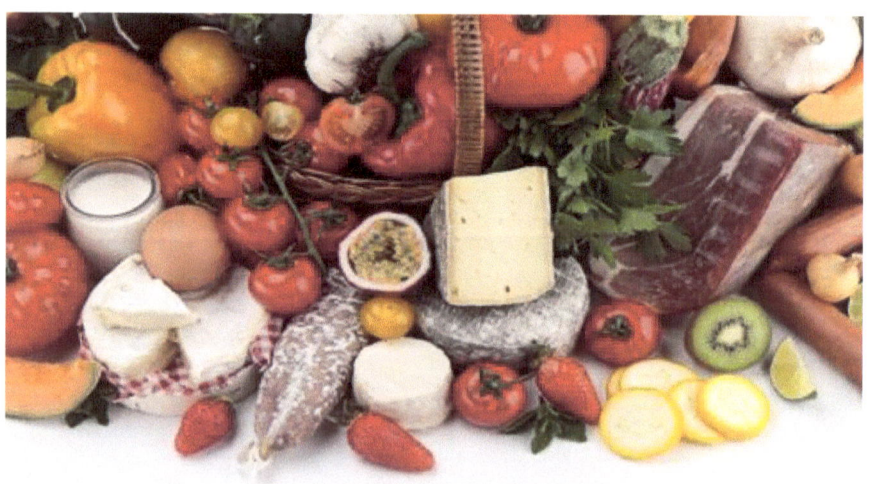

Image credit:123RF Stock

A "healthy diet" has become a bit of a catch phrase in recent decades. It seems that you can't turn on the television or even read a magazine without seeing advertisements for fad diets, weight loss supplements, and other products that promise rapid weight loss. While these things may work for the short-term, they rarely lead to long-term success. If you have a few pounds to lose or you are at the beginning of a long weight loss journey, it is important to be patient with your body and avoid the temptation of fad dieting. Instead treat your body kindly and fill it with healthy foods with a reasonable balance of water, carbs, fat, protein, and sugar.

Although this may seem like a simple concept to put into motion, the truth is that it can be hard to eat a balanced diet, especially with so much misinformation being touted as truth. For instance, in the past several years it has become generally accepted that a low-fat or fat-free diet is the healthiest. This concept has been widely adopted by society as the "norm" for a healthy lifestyle. It has also been a source of marketing in the food industry, with marketers putting "fat free" on food labels – even those that never had fat to begin with!

The initial trend in fat-free diets and products was due to the fact that the science and research at the time was correlating high fat diets to increased risk of heart disease. This led to a lot of the big food companies trying to stay on trend by creating fat-free or low-fat food products. The issue that arose was that once you removed the fat from food products they ended up not tasting as good to the consumer.To assure that products kept their delicious taste, food companies resorted to adding another great tasting macronutrient to their products. Can you guess what this delicious and sweet nutrient was? If you guessed sugar, you would be right!

Companies created fat-free products that still tasted delicious, but were in turn packed full of added sugar. They added sugar to everything...soups, breads, crackers, canned fruits and vegetables, yogurt, and even milk. This trend in food production is a very large contributing factor to the current obesity epidemic.

What you may or may notrealize about sugar consumption is that when sugar is quickly absorbed into the blood stream the body is forced to store the excess energy as fat. The key here is that sugar turns to fat as soon as it hits your system. When you stop to consider this it becomes quite obvious why obesity have become such a major problem for a large percentage of the population.

More recent studies are emerging which indicate that diets high in fat may not be as harmful to our heart as we once thought. Although having high cholesterol and fat in your system can be damaging, current trends in research demonstrate that it is the high amounts of sugar that are actually initiating the physiological processes responsible for heart disease.

Restricting the amount of calories consumed is often a

strategy people believe will make them healthier. This idea exists in people's minds because they associate calorie restriction with maintaining weight and they in turn associate maintaining weight with being healthy. This concept isn't totally wrong as being the proper weight for your height and age is important for overall health. The mistake people are making is putting too much stake in the concept that calories consumed must equal calories expended to maintain weight and be healthy. This statement over simplifies the body's metabolic processes and how your system breaks down and uses energy. More emphasis should be placed on what you're eating instead of how many calories you're consuming.

If focus was placed more on eating whole foods consisting primarily of vegetables, healthy fats,and lean meats, our bodies would respond with a consistently balanced blood sugar and insulin level, as well as a more stable physiological state. Overall wellness and a healthy weight would simply fall into place and there wouldn't be as many people worried about their lack of energy.

What does this mean for you? It means you can relax and stop counting calories. That, in and of itself, can be exhausting and waste a lot of energy. Instead eat healthy, whole foods as part of a balanced diet and eat as much as you want! Your body will thank you for it and in return will give you endless energy, an enhanced mood, a lean body and an overall feeling of boundless well-being.

At Pinewood Natural Health Centre, we focus on diet and

nutrition as part of every patient's treatment plan as the cornerstone of long-term health success by establishing small, attainable goals to guide you to a state of optimal health and wellness. Not only do we focus on the solid foods that are going into your body, but we address the liquids you are consuming as well.

Would it surprise you to learn that people consume more soda, juice, coffee, and other drinks, but not one of the easiest and cheapest liquids – water? Water is the most important nutrient for our bodies, just as important for survival as oxygen. Yet it is often dismissed for tastier, flavorful drinks that provide very little nutrition to our bodies.

Why do we need water? The human body loses approximately 2.4 liters of water every day, so replenishing that lost supply is vital our health. Water assists in every body system – digestion, regulation of body temperature, blood circulation, ensuring cells in the body receive nutrients and oxygen, removing toxins, joint movement, and metabolism of stored fats, maintenance of muscle tone, and much more. Getting enough water ensures that all systems of the body work together effectively.

Finally, research has revealed that food intolerances can have dramatic effects on our health. Food intolerances occur when the body has difficulty assimilating some component of food. It can be diary, wheat, gluten, and more. Food intolerance can manifest in a variety of symptoms; diarrhea and other abdominal symptoms, rashes and itching, weight gain and bloating, and more.

All of these factors; diet, water consumption and food intolerance directly affects the amount of energy we have. A diet too high in sugar or fat can cause sluggishness and lack of energy. Not enough water can lead to headaches, achiness and lethargy. Food intolerances cause us to feel sick and generally unwell, leading to low energy levels.

The fix – Find more balance

The proper balance between fruit, vegetables, meats, fat, and sugar results in optimum nutrition. A balanced diet provides the optimal level of calories we need to maintain our energy levels and provide fuel for our bodies. The following is the average daily recommended food servings for adults, per Health Canada.

Vegetables and Fruit: 7 servings

Grain Products: 7 servings*

Milk and Alternatives: 3 servings

Meat and Alternatives: 3 servings

Oils and Fats: 2-3 tablespoons of unsaturated fat

*In cases where a patient is trying to manage their weight, seven servings of grain products may be too high. At Pinewood Natural Health Centre, we work with our patients to develop a nutritional plan that takes into account the overall health and wellness goals of our patients. The food serving recommendations above should only be used as a guideline.Below is a chart adapted from Health Canada, which provides more detailed guidelines for a healthy diet.

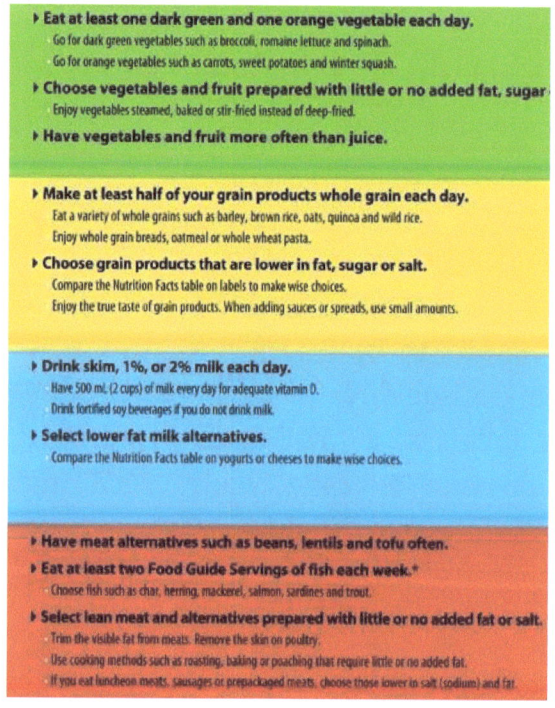

The additional benefit to a healthy diet is consumption of all necessary vitamins and minerals. A balanced diet should provide all the vitamins and minerals you need to maintain a healthy lifestyle.

It is generally accepted that it's important to eat breakfast, eat a larger, healthy lunch, and don't overdo it at dinner. Your body needs more energy in the first part of the day, so it makes more sense to consume more healthy calories at the beginning of the day. Skipping breakfast makes you hungrier during the day, increasing the likelihood that you will overeat later. There is still some debate over whether it's better to eat three square meals or to eat more frequent, smaller meals throughout the day; however as long as you're getting the recommended amount of fruits and veggies, you should be well on your way to a healthy, balanced diet. In the end, the number of meals you eat throughout the day may simply be a personal preference. What is best for one person may not fit into your lifestyle. Diet and nutrition is not necessarily one-size-fits-all.

Experts also hesitate to recommend a specific number when talking about water consumption. Generally, the recommendation is eight glasses a day, primarily because it is easy to remember. The most important thing to know is that you should drink enough water that you never begin to feel the signs of dehydration. Generally, this means not feeling thirsty and urinating frequently throughout the day. Also remember that if you're exercising, live in a hot environment, are sick or pregnant or breastfeeding, you will need to consume more water than the average adult.

Starting your day off by consuming two glasses of warm water will not only help you stay hydrated and feeling alert (dehydration can cause your body to feel tired), but it will also help you kick-start your water consumption for the day. Ideally, everyone should aim to drink at least half of their body weight in water each day. If you prefer flavor, consider adding the juice of half a lemon to your water. Lemons are considered an alkaline food, which is considered a key to good health.

Are you in control of your food intolerances?

Addressing your food intolerances instead of ignoring them or resigning to the notion that you will just have to "live with it" is crucial if you want to reboot your energy. Lactose, a sugar which is found in diary and milk products, is a common type of food intolerance. Other intolerances include gluten, sulfites, and other food additives. People that have food intolerances usually experience symptoms when they eat too much of a certain type of food. These symptoms include:

- Nausea

- Cramping

- Diarrhea

- Vomiting

It is important to recognize the difference between food intolerances, a food allergy, and food sensitivities. Many people use these terms interchangeably and although they may share symptoms, there are differences that people need to be aware of to find the best treatment.

Food allergies do not come and go. Symptoms occur every time you encounter or ingest that particular food. Symptoms such as shortness of breath, hives, chest pains, and in some cases, a sudden drop in blood pressure come on suddenly. A person experiencing a food allergy does not have to eat a lot of the food item to break out in a rash or experience other symptoms such as shortness of breath, chest pains, or, in some cases, a sudden drop in blood pressure. Food allergies, unlike food intolerances, are something that can be life-threatening and should be avoided.

At Pinewood Natural Health Centre, your doctor can help you determine if you have food intolerances, sensitivities, or food allergies. Keeping a food journal is one way that medical professionals diagnose food intolerances. By recording the types of foods you eat, the amount of the serving, the frequency of ingestions, and how your body physically reacts after consuming these foods, you and your doctor will be able to discover patterns that can shed light on the situation.

Patients that are diagnosed with food intolerances are generally advised to avoid certain foods or eat smaller portions to avoid unpleasant symptoms that can leave you feeling drained of energy. In cases of food sensitivity, a person is generally affected by certain foods even though no known medical reason exists for the negative symptoms. If food sensitivity is suspected, then the patient may be advised to participate in an elimination diet, avoiding the foods that make them ill and then participate in a challenge phase where the foods are introduced back into the diet a little at a time to determine if tolerance is something that can be achieved.

What's Zapping Your Energy?

The doctors at Pinewood Natural Health Centre work with individuals presenting a variety of food related intolerances, sensitivities, and allergies on a daily basis. These are issues that should be taken seriously because they are more than a pain. Eating the wrong foods for your body can actually lessen the quality of your life and create chronic pain that could be avoided.

Vitamins – A Supplemental Form of Energy

Your body needs a certain amount of vitamins each day to ward off exhaustion, illness and disease. Ideally, these nutritional needs should be met by eating a well-balanced diet full of whole grains, fruits and vegetables. But for the majority of people, acquiring their daily dose of vitamins in this manner can be rather difficult. From confusion over labels to poor food quality, eating healthy to acquire your daily dose of vitamins isn't always so cut and dry. This is why vitamins or dietary supplements make sense to meet your daily needs.

Complete nutrition should never come in a bottle, but there are benefits to taking a daily multi-vitamin. The vitamins and minerals in a multi-vitamin can boost your immune system, fight fatigue, improve brain function, assist with digestion, and may even shift hormonal balances responsible for the aging process, resulting in a happier, healthier, younger feeling you!

Mistake #2: Your Emotions are Exhausting
The problem: Negative thoughts and emotions drain energy

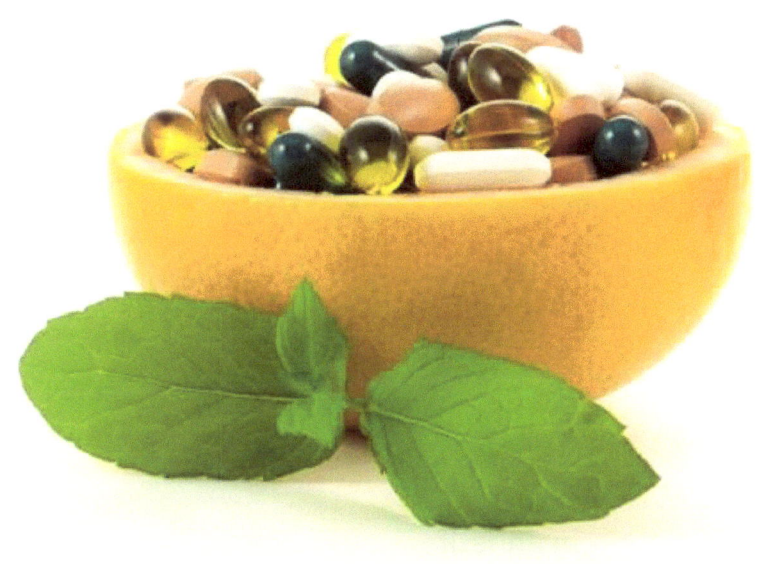

Image credit:123RF Stock

What's Zapping Your Energy?

Have you ever heard someone say, "It takes more muscles to frown than it does to smile?" While it may not be scientifically sound, it can't be argued that when we're happy, we feel better. When we're sad, angry, anxious, or scared, we don't feel well. It's exhausting to be unhappy.

When we don't feel well physically, we get tired. Research shows that negative thoughts cause our thinking to become narrow and shut off the world around you. You become isolated, increasing your negative feelings, and it becomes a cycle. Given long enough, those negative thoughts will manifest into physical symptoms:

- Headaches

- Chest pain

- Digestive problems

- Back pain

- Muscle and joint pain

- Changes in appetite

- Exhaustion and fatigue

And we all know that being uncomfortable or in pain makes you tired.

The fix: The power of positive thinking

It's important that you are able to identify the reasons

you're feeling sad or anxious, so that you can begin to seek help. If there is something negative happening in your life – a divorce, loss of work, or a death in the family, it can cause us to feel sad and anxious for a period of time – known as situational depression. Sadness can also manifest as Seasonal Affective Disorder, which happens in the winter months, where some people have a difficult time with less sunlight and time outdoors.

Chronic depression is a medical condition, caused by chemicals in the brain that aren't properly balanced. If you suspect you're suffering from depression, it's important that you seek help. Not only does depression make you tired, it can also become a serious threat to your health. Signs of chronic depression include:

1. Persistent sad, anxious, or "empty" mood

2. Feelings of hopelessness or pessimism

3. Feelings of guilt, worthlessness, or helplessness

4. Loss of interest or pleasure in hobbies and activities that were once enjoyed, including sex

5. Decreased energy, fatigue, or feeling "slowed down"

6. Difficulty concentrating, remembering, or making decisions

7. Insomnia, early-morning awakening, or oversleeping

8. Appetite and/or weight loss or overeating and weight gain

9. Thoughts of death or suicide or actual suicide attempts

10. Restlessness or irritability

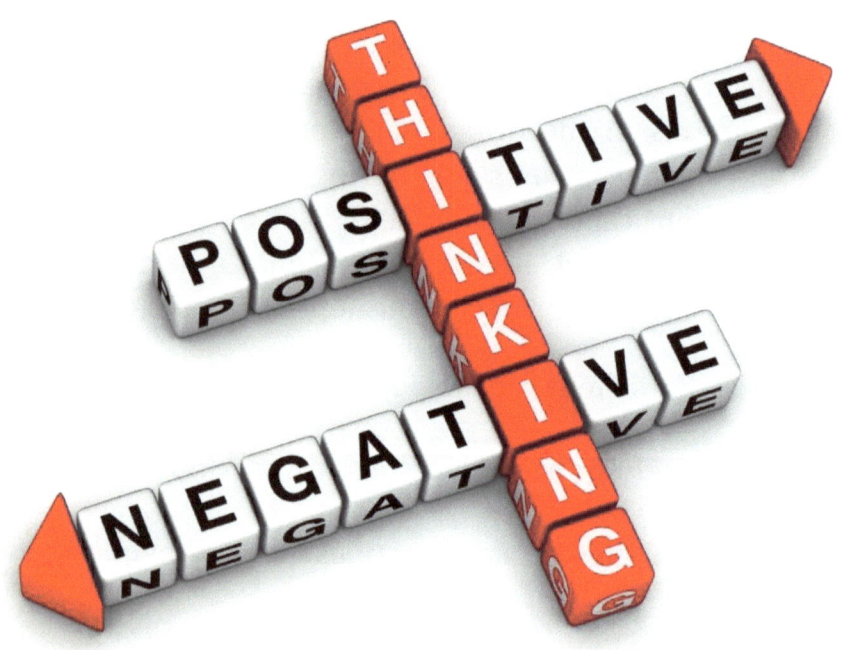

Image credit: 123RF Stock Photo

What if you're not suffering from depression but still find yourself thinking negative thoughts? Some people are, by nature, pessimistic, but negative thinking has a huge impact on your health. In addition to many of the same physical symptoms seen with depression, thinking negatively can impact your work and relationships with family and friends.

Studies show that positive thinking directly impacts the way we feel. Positive thinkers tend to cope better with stress, which can greatly influence one's overall health. Individuals that choose to look at life with a "glass half full" attitude tend to be resistant to disease, reduce their chances of developing cardiovascular problems, have fewer depressive episodes, and tend to achieve higher life expectancy rates.

Positive thinking isn't about ignoring negative influences in your life. It is about looking at a situation from all angles and choosing to be resilient; to find resolution, pick up the pieces and move forward in life. People that have a pessimistic attitude tend to exert all their energy wallowing in their own despair. This negative outlook is not conducive to a healthy lifestyle and can wear a person down psychologically and physiologically at a rapid pace.

How can you conjure positivity in your life? The first step is removing the interference between your body and the power that created your physical being.

Your emotions and thoughts are directly connected to your physical well-being. Take a moment to test out this theory. Think about something that is unpleasant. That brings about sad or uncomfortable memories. Now pay attention to how your body reacts to these thoughts. Maybe your heart quickens or you feel a slight pounding behind your temples. Next, think of a happy memory;

something that made you feel safe, relaxed and joyful. How does your body react to these thoughts? Has your breathing slowed? Is your heart rate steady? These are clear examples of the mind/body connection and how your thoughts shape your physical well-being.

Living healthy is more than just eating the right foods, getting the right amount of exercise, and staying away from toxins like alcohol and cigarettes. It is about understanding that you have the power within you to ward off the physical ramifications that negative thoughts and energy can do to your body. Once you make the mind/body connection and started focusing your thoughts in the right direction, you will begin to experience vitality once again.

One way to foster the mind/body connection is to introduce spiritual practices such as breathing, meditation and/or visualization. These are tools that you have at your disposal every moment to aid you in achieving self-awareness, focusing the mind and inviting positive energy into your life. Incorporating these practices into your daily life not only has physical side effects, but it can improve your emotional health.

If meditation and visualization is something completely new to you, start off slowly. To begin, abandon all expectations. These practices are entirely personal. No one person experiences the same sensations as another and your experience may be different with each new session. For beginners, box breathing or four squared breathing is a wonderful way to incorporate deep breathing practices into your everyday life.

Box breathing is ideal for reducing stress. It is controlled breathing designed to minimize anxiety and calm your nerves. It can be used alone or with meditation and visualization practices. First, find a comfortable place to sit that is free from distractions. The room should be quiet with dim lighting for maximum benefits. You can sit either in a chair or seated on the floor. Make sure your posture is aligned and that you are at ease. Once you are seated comfortably, breathe in the following manner:

1. Breathe in through your nose counting to four as you inhale. Next hold your breath for four counts.

2. Release the air slowly through your mouth this time counting to four as you exhale and hold the exhale for four counts.

It is recommended that you continue to breath in this manner for a minimum of four minutes; however, boxed breathing can be quite effective at calming the nerves in immediate situations when the entire cycle is practiced just two or three times.

Boxed breathing brings the respiratory system back into alignment and stops shallow breathing that often accompanies stress, fear, and pain.

Practitioners use the boxed breathing techniques as well as other meditation and visualization practices such as deliberate imagination and mountain top awareness to assist the subconscious in meeting the conscious. These mind/body practices have a dramatic effect on the nervous system that can drastically change your outlook on life and your physical well-being.

Mistake #3: You Exercise too Little – or too Much

The problem: Your exercise patterns aren't healthy

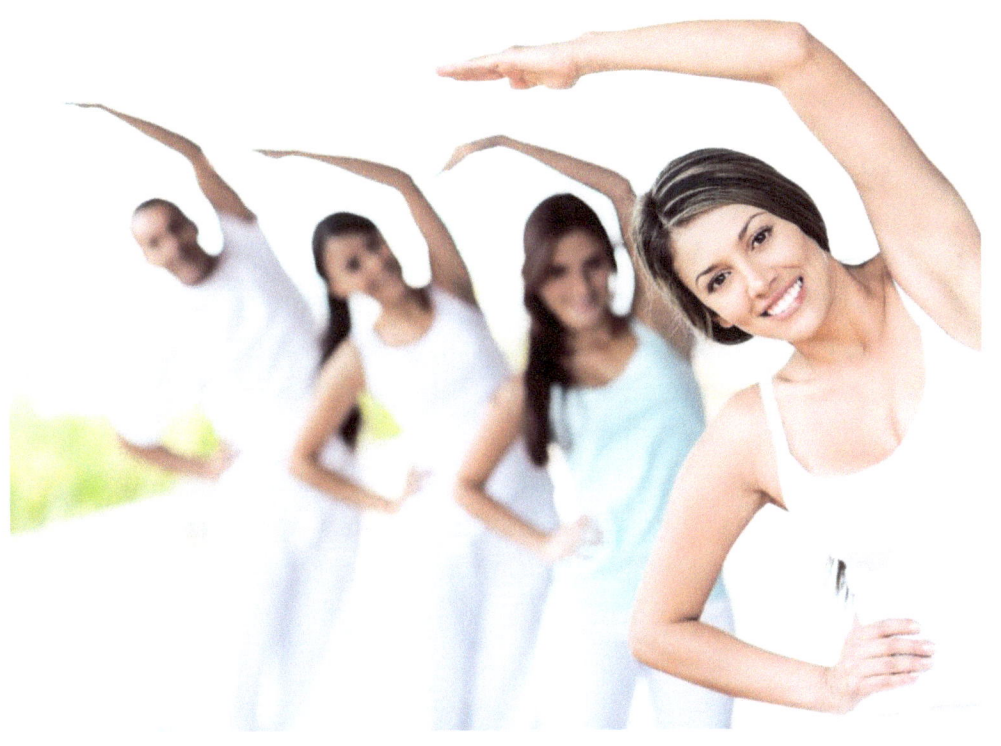

Image credit:123RF Stock Photo

What's Zapping Your Energy?

There are countless benefits to healthy exercise habits. Exercise can help you maintain a healthy weight, improve cardiovascular and digestive health, it can aid in preventing osteoporosis, warding off certain cancers, and help you avoid depression and anxiety. Quite honestly the list goes on and on and is too extensive to list every single benefit! Most importantly, exercise helps us sleep better, leaving us feeling well-rested and restored.

But what happens when your exercise patterns aren't healthy?

If you don't exercise at all, you are at risk for unhealthy weight gain, which can lead to high blood pressure, type 2 diabetes, and heart problems. A sedentary lifestyle can also be attributed to muscle atrophy, the decrease of muscle mass that can lead to complete or partial wasting away of the muscles in one's body. As you age, your muscles need to be continuously strengthened to combat this condition. You don't need to lift hundreds of pounds or build up a physique that resembles a body builder. Simple, daily exercise that includes cardiovascular and strengthening sessions will keep your muscles in top form.

Brittle bones and decreased bone density are additional problems that face the aging population in regards to exercise. The bones in your body will naturally lose density with each additional candle that you blow out on your birthday cake each year, but that doesn't mean that you can't fight back and battle against brittle bones and conditions like osteoporosis. Weight-bearing exercises can strengthen your bones, reducing your chances of broken bones and degenerating conditions.

Are there dangers of exercising too much?

Absolutely! As with anything in life, you have to find balance. People that overexert themselves or take fitness to the extreme are at risk for developing overuse injuries, chronic pain, dehydration, and unhealthy weight loss. Most people do not set out to overexert themselves when exercising. In many cases, it happens because the person assumes their body is reacting to the increased cardiovascular state. For this reason, it is important that if you are new to exercising or you have changed your current routine that you stay alert to signs of overexertion such as:

- Rapid heart rate

- Nausea

- Stomach pains

- Headaches

- Weakness

- Excessive tiredness

If you have a heart condition, respiratory problems, or another condition that requires the continual attention of a physician, it is important to speak with them before beginning any exercise routine to avoid life-threatening circumstances.

The fix: Find out what is healthy exercise for your age and body type

Regular exercise reduces your changes of chronic illnesses, while improving your total health and fitness. But how much should you be exercising? According to the Canadian Society for Exercise Physiology (CSEP), adults between the ages of 18 and 64 should strive to achieve 150 minutes (just under two hours) of moderate to dynamic physical activity each week. For muscle and bone strengthening, the general recommendation is to engage in activities that focus on strengthening the major muscles groups at least two times per week.

The goal is to simply stay in motion. You can attain a reasonable amount of fitness by merely changing your habits. For example, you can take the stairs instead of the elevator or you can park farther away from the entrance to your office. Incorporating after dinner walks or walking first thing in the morning not only keeps you in physical shape, but it can be a great way to unwind or prepare for your day.

When it comes to exercise, you have many options depending on your physical abilities, your available time, and your overall fitness goals. For cardiovascular endurance, many people choose jogging or walking. This is a simple way to add regular exercise into your daily routine and can be done anywhere, anytime, and doesn't require any special equipment other than a good pair of athletic shoes.

If you have bad knees or problems with your joints, you may want to avoid high impact activities like jogging or running and, instead, stick with walking briskly or consider other low impact options such as: swimming, hiking, biking, or using a machine like the elliptical. Although you may burn more calories faster with high impact options, low impact activities are just as effective at helping you achieve your exercise goals, while increasing your energy.

Whether you engage in high or low impact cardiovascular activities, it is crucial that your routine includes a stretching sequence. Stretching is therapeutic to your body. Not only does it warm your body up when preparing for vigorous exercise, but when incorporated regularly into your lifestyle it can elongate your muscles, increase your flexibility, and boost your range of motion reducing injuries and soothing chronic pain.

Our bodies endure a lot of stress throughout the day. Even if you are not engaging in full-out exercise, simply moving about puts wear and tear on your body; your joints and your muscles. A body that is stagnant or inflexible will tire more easily when performing normal, everyday activities. Something as simple as bending over and tying your shoes, can leave you feeling tight and exhausted.

By adding a stretching sequence into your daily routine,

you will feel younger and have more energy. Stretching can also help you achieve the mind/body connection that is crucial for overall health and wellness. As you continue to incorporate stretches into your daily life, you will become more aware of your body's movements and your breath. This awareness helps you achieve that mind/body connection, reducing stress and anxiety that often contributes to exhaustion.

The Sun Salutation is a series of yoga stretches that are straightforward and easy for anyone to do. You can do this series in the morning when you wake up or do it before bed to help you relax. You may even choose to do it to bookend your days. Sun Salutation consists of 12 poses that are done in a graceful flow, while concentrating on fluid, consistent breathing. There are various sites online that demonstrate the flow or your doctor at Pinewood Natural Health Centre can provide you with instruction.

Mistake #4: You're Not Getting Enough Sleep
The problem: Life is busy and you're not making sleep a priority

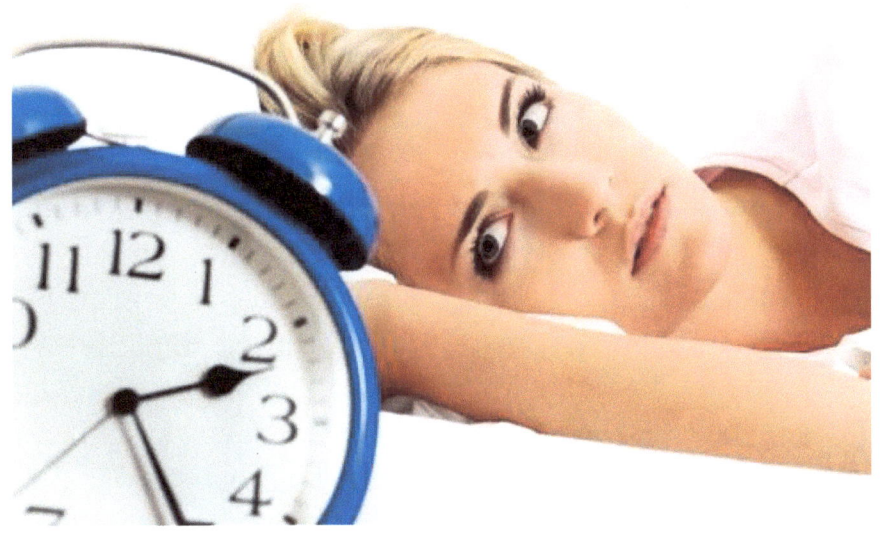

Image credit: 123RF Stock Photo

What's Zapping Your Energy?

Are you turning the sheets back later and later because you are trying to get too much done at night and choosing to sacrifice sleep? Perhaps you are having a difficult time managing your thoughts, finding yourself lying awake for hours every night making mental lists of what needs to be done the next day. With the demands of work, family, and schedules that are packed full with extracurricular activities, finding time to sleep and being able to actually fall asleep once your head hits the pillow can be nearly impossible. What are you to do? Give in and add an extra dose or two of caffeine to your morning espresso?

Although many people manage their exhaustion in this manner, it is not a long-term solution. The best solution is to recognize your sleep patterns are unhealthy and take action to develop healthy sleep patterns that leave you feeling well rested without being tempted to hit the snooze button each morning. The first step is figuring out what is causing your sleep to be disrupted. Sometimes it is as simple as reducing your workload or rearranging your schedule, but there are other factors that can contribute to shifting sleep patterns such as:

- Age – As you age, you have less uninterrupted sleep and fewer REM episodes. These episodes should comprise 20 to 25 percent of an entire night's sleep in healthy adults. If you used to dream and have suddenly stopped dreaming, you may want to consult with a sleep specialist.

- Stress – This is one of the main reasons that contribute to restless nights. Learning how to manage your stress is mission critical. Delegating responsibilities, practicing time management, and even engaging in meditative practices can help you calm your body to prepare it for a restful night's sleep.

- Exercise – Engaging in physical fitness before bedtime can make it difficult to fall asleep. While your body may be exhausted from a vigorous routine, that doesn't mean that you will be able to fall asleep quickly. Ideally, you want to exercise several hours before bedtime.

- Temperature – If you are having problems sleeping, it could be that your bedroom is too cold or too hot. Because your body experiences a mild drop in body temperature when you sleep, the temperature that is just right while you are awake may be too hot or cold while you sleep. While it is difficult to come up with a recommended range for sleeping because every person is different, the ideal temperature range for bedtime is between 20 and 23 degrees Celsius.

- Light – When a room is too bright, the body's internal clock may get the time of day confused, resulting in premature wakefulness. Ideally, you should sleep without lights on. If you are a shift worker and must sleep during the day, consider purchasing black-out blinds or shades to reduce the amount of natural light filtering into your bedroom.

- Medications – Certain medications can affect your sleep patterns, too. If you are taking medications and notice you are waking more often throughout the night or having difficulty falling asleep, consider speaking with your physician to determine if there are other medications you could take or if you could take the prescription several hours before bedtime.

- Non-traditional work hours – Shift workers and those with varying schedules may have an extremely difficult time getting the deep, restful sleep they need. If adjusting your schedule is not possible, speak with your physician to determine if there are supplements or other natural remedies that may help you achieve the sleep your body requires.

Lastly, don't confuse quality of sleep with quantity of sleep. When you toss and turn throughout the night and wake up every two or three hours, you are not getting quality sleep. If you are struggling to stay asleep during the night, it's time to take action.

The fix: Overhaul your sleep patterns

How much sleep does the average person need? On average, adults need between seven and nine hours of sleep each night. Unfortunately, most adults only manage to get six or fewer hours of sleep. With so many people finding it difficult to attain the recommended number of hours for sleep, it is no wonder that a major complaint among adults is that they feel run-down and excessively tired day in and day out.

Luckily, sleep deprivation is something that is easily correctable – that is when you make time for sleep. Like many things in life, we have to make a conscious effort to maintain healthy sleep habits. By clearing your schedule, saying "no" to taking on one more project at work, or slimming down your family's activity schedule, you can create more hours in your day. When you do this, you can find the time you need to be in bed each night at a reasonable hour. As you can see, it's not a magical solution, merely a practical solution that has an enormous impact on your physical and emotional well-being.

Do you know the benefits of healthy sleep cycles?

There are a number of benefits that extend beyond simply feeling refreshed and alert. In fact, people that ignore the importance of establishing healthy sleep cycles are not only putting themselves at risk, but the people around them, too. Activities like driving can be dangerous to the general public when you are sleep deprived. If you work in an industry where other people's well-being depends on you, such as in the medical field, you could put another person's life in jeopardy if you are overtired. Machine operators, over-the-road truck drivers, air traffic control operators, pilots, cab drivers, bus drivers – these are just a handful of examples of people that could negatively impact others as a result of not getting enough sleep.

When you make it a priority to practice healthy sleep habits, your body will respond in a positive manner. By sticking to a bedtime routine and getting the recommended hours of sleep each night, you will:

- Be more alert

- Feel energetic

- Increase your memory

- Reduce delayed reactions to external stimuli

- Be able to multi-task efficiently

- Feel happier

In addition to the listed benefits, you will reduce your chances of cardiovascular disease, increase your immunity and your hormones will stay in balance. To live a vibrant, healthy lifestyle, you have to make sleep a priority. It really is just that simple.

Are you managing your sleep hygiene?

You take care of your body in a number of ways. You practice daily oral hygiene, you eat the right types of foods and you exercise an appropriate amount; all of these habits are essential to maintaining a high level of health and wellness. But what about taking care of your sleep hygiene? Are you doing everything you can do to promote healthier, better sleep for you? The best way to determine if your sleep hygiene needs to be tweaked is to ask yourself the following questions:

- Do I adhere to a strict bedtime?

- Do I "sleep in" on the weekends?

- Have I created a peaceful sleep environment that is free from other distractions?

- Am I feeling the urge to nap frequently throughout the day?

Bedtimes are not just for young children. Adults can benefit from regular bedtimes, too. The human body thrives on routine, which is regulated by your sleep and wake times. Irregular sleep patterns can throw the body off. It can disrupt hormonal balances, affect your mood, and reduce your body's ability to naturally fight off infections. While sleeping in on the weekends may be your way of catching up on your sleep, falling into this habit can actually make you more tired. It is better to follow a strict sleep schedule, seven days a week, without any variance. Of course, there will be times when this is difficult due to events or other engagements, but making it a priority the majority of the time to get to bed on time and wake up at the same time each morning will go a long way in helping you feel less exhausted, allowing you to feel refreshed and robust each day.

What's Zapping Your Energy?

Following a bedtime schedule isn't the only aspect of a well-rounded sleep hygiene routine. Creating a peaceful sleep environment is central to falling asleep quickly and deeply. Your bedroom should be a place of utter relaxation free from distractions like smart/cell phones, tablets, televisions, and other gadgets that encourage alertness instead of restful relaxation. By refusing to make your bedroom a multi-purpose room, you will reduce both physical and mental clutter that can make it hard to fall asleep and stay asleep.

Did you know that the sleep cycle actually begins before you fall asleep? Shortly before our habitual bedtime, our bodies begin to secrete the hormone melatonin. This starts the psychological process associated with falling asleep. You can naturally encourage the release of melatonin by reducing the amount of light in your bedroom and in other rooms in your house prior to retiring to bed. For instance, if you are watching television, about 30 minutes before you decide to turn in for the night, turn down the lights. Bright lights prohibit the release of melatonin, making it harder to make the transition from wakefulness to sleep.

If you wake up in the middle of the night to use the bathroom or get a drink of water, resist the temptation to turn on the lights. Circadian rhythms are greatly affected by external stimuli, especially light. This can make it hard to fall back asleep once you return to bed. Using nightlights to illuminate the path to your bathroom or to the kitchen will provide you with enough light without disrupting melatonin production and throwing off your circadian rhythm.

Lastly, another way to avoid disrupting your body's natural circadian rhythm is to avoid napping during the day. When napping becomes a habit, you fragment your sleep. This fragmentation can make it hard to fall asleep at its best, but at its worst it can lead to insomnia. If a nap is unavoidable, make it a short nap. Avoid naps that extend past 15 – 20 minutes.

Mistake #5: Hormones are Wreaking Havoc on Your Body
The problem: Your hormones are out of balance

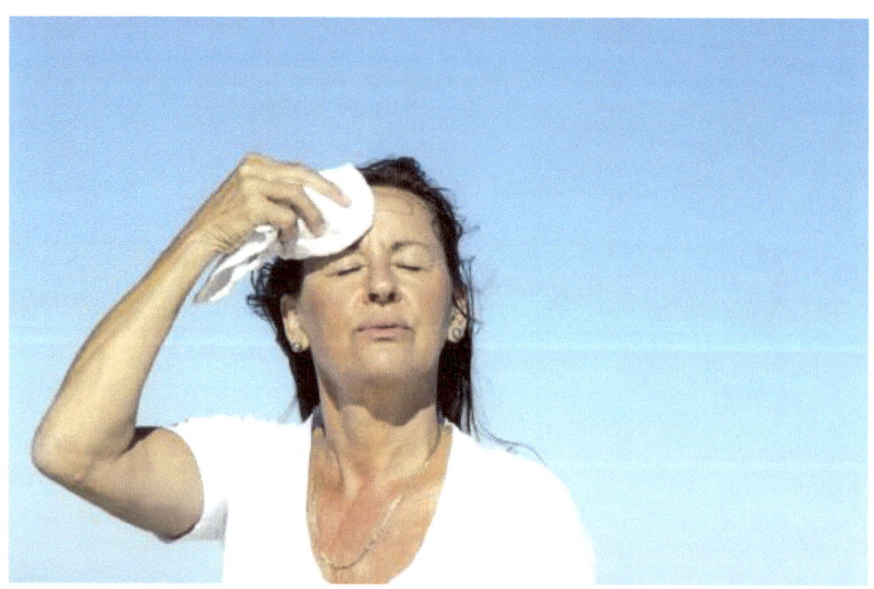

Image credit:123RF Stock Photo

Mistake #5: Hormones are Wreaking Havoc on Your Body

Feeling stressed out? When you are feeling overwhelmed and at your wits end, these feelings aren't just in your head. Or, are they?

The human brain produces a stress hormone callednoradrenalin. The brain releases this hormone into the blood stream when a person feels stress, danger, or is even just a tad bit frazzled. Once this hormone makes its way into your bloodstream, physical side effects like an increased heart rate and a spike in energy occur. The body is conditioned to deal with a certain amount of stress thanks to this particular hormone; however, when your stress levels rise beyond normal limits the brain, due to negative inhibition, actually inhibits the body from moving the cortisol through the bloodstream, resulting in too little cortisol. This actually represents adrenal fatigue. The effects of this reaction will leave a person feeling spent and wondering why they all of a sudden feel like they were ran over by a train.

Stress can also trigger unbalanced hormonal releases from the thyroid and adrenal glands. Your body's thyroid gland regulates your metabolism and contributes to your energy levels. When you are under a great deal of stress, struggling with nutritional deficiencies, or even experiencing chronic inflammation due to conditions like arthritis, your thyroid gland will react by leaving you feeling fatigued.

Low levels of melatonin can also lead to excessive tiredness and lack of energy. Melatonin is produced in a small area of the brain known as the pineal gland.

Melatonin naturally controls the body's sleep cycle. When your body doesn't produce the correct amounts of melatonin it can affect your ability to fall asleep or stay asleep. This hormone is produced naturally by the body, but can also be found in very small amounts in certain foods. Foods that have niacinamide, vitamin B-6, calcium and magnesium are best for generating more of this sleep aid hormone.

As you age, your body will produce lesser amounts of melatonin. You can counteract the effects of aging by consulting with your doctor at Pinewood Natural Health Centre about natural ways to increase your melatonin production.

The fix: Get your hormones back in balance

Bioidentical Hormones

Lately, many women – and even some men – are discovering the revolutionary wonder in the advancement of bioidentical hormones. Bioidentical hormones are referred to as natural hormone therapy or bioidentical hormone replacement therapy (BHRT). BHRT may sound complicated and atypical, but this therapy is defined as hormones that are identical to the hormones naturally produced in an individual's body.

There are a number of different types of bioidentical hormones such as: bioidentical estrogen, bioidentical progesterone, bioidentical testosterone, etc. For women, in particular, the loss of estrogen can be something that throws their body out of balance as they approach and go through menopause. Post-menopausal women experience a decrease of estrogen that can lead to severe symptoms such as fatigue, loss of sex drive, weight gain, and so forth. By utilizing BHRT the estrogen hormone can be replaced. Because the molecular biology of the bioidentical hormones mimics natural hormones, the body cannot tell the difference between the natural and the bioidentical hormone.

What are the benefits of BHRT? Women and men that use this therapy to replace estrogen, progesterone, or testosterone, report a better quality of life and anti-aging relief. One of the great things about BHRT is that not only can they be administered by a doctor, but they can also be found naturally in every day foods such as yams and soy products. What does this mean for you? It means that you can replenish your hormones naturally when your body stops producing them in excess by choosing hormone friendly foods that are abundant and easily incorporated into your diet.

At Pinewood Natural Health Centre, patients receive customized BHRT by administering individualized natural hormone therapy using blood hormone testing. This individualized testing enables the doctors to fine tune your hormone therapy to avoid unpleasant side-effects or health risks. Pinewood Natural Health Centre offers comprehensive BHRT clinical packages allowing you and your doctor to make the best therapeutic decisions to meet your body's individual needs.

What's Zapping Your Energy?

BHRT is designed to help you feel like yourself again after significant hormonal changes. However, BHRT may not be for everyone. Bioidentical hormones have been known to contribute to certain medical problems such as cardiovascular disease, heart attack, or stroke. This is why it is crucial that you receive an individual analysis of your situation to determine if natural hormone replacement therapies are a healthy, safe option for you.

Why Choose Pinewood?

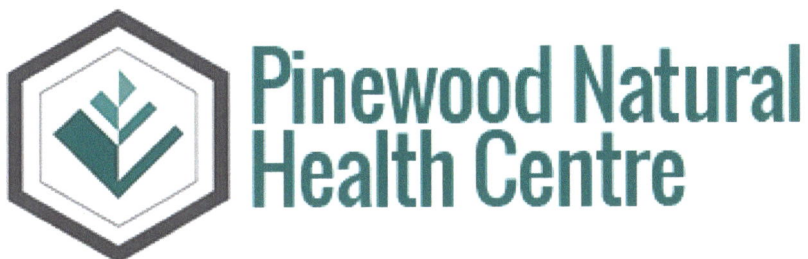

What's Zapping Your Energy?

Since 1997, our clinic has helped thousands of patients just like you overcome nagging health issues, increase energy, reduce stress, and dramatically improve their quality of life. We'd love the opportunity to help you too. The beauty of our approach is that we utilize a variety of proven, natural healthcare methods to optimize your healing process. The combination of therapies and methods we use creates a synergistic and profound level of benefit for our patients.

Right now, you may be feeling overwhelmed or frustrated with your healthcare choices. Perhaps you've tried conventional medicine and it isn't capable of treating the root cause of your health concerns. You also know the degree to which stress impacts your health, and you're looking for gentle yet effective ways to calm your mind and clear your stress while improving your physical health. This is where we excel and can help you in a way that few other clinics can!

At Pinewood Natural Health Centre, we take a multi-disciplinary approach to treating our patients. Using an integrated system of medicine, we use holistic healing practices to prevent and treat disease to help our patients obtain optimal health benefits. Our mission at Pinewood is to support and encourage our patients to maintain their overall health and wellness, while teaching responsible self-healing and always providing the highest standards of superior professional patient care.

We treat our patients as individuals selecting therapies

and treatments that will address individual needs. We offer our patients a wide variety of naturopathic options based on their symptoms, current medical conditions, and their healing goals. Examples of our therapies and treatments include:

- Botanical Medicine

- Homeopathy

- Traditional Chinese Medicine and Acupuncture

- Stress Management and Lifestyle Counselling

- Clinical Nutrition

- Physical Modalities

At Pinewood, all of our treatment plans are fully individualized. No two people are alike; therefore, no two treatments are ever the same.

If you are tired of dealing with chronic pain, fatigue, stress, or general lifestyle imbalances and want to infuse energy and vitality back into your life, then give us a call at (416) 656-8100 or visit our website www.pinewoodhealth.ca to learn more about how Pinewood Natural Health Centre can profoundly impact your lifestyle.

We offer complimentary naturopathic visits for first time patients so you can learn about our methods and make an informed decision about your treatment plan. Our doctors and staff are committed to providing you with exceptional, individualized care so that you can live the life you were meant to live!

Our Practitioners and Team
Dr. Michael Rahman, BSc, ND

Dr. Rahman completed his Bachelor of Science with an emphasis on biology at McMaster University in 1993. He furthered his studies at the Canadian College of Naturopathic Medicine and completed a four year doctorate program in Toronto. He is licensed to practice in both Ontario and British Columbia. His practice focuses on biological medicine and its treatment of chronic diseases, from fibromyalgia to cancer, and healthy age management. His practice interest also includes naturopathic cosmetic care, blending naturopathic medicine with cosmetic approaches and technology to enhance health and beauty.

Dr. Rahmam is an active member of the Ontario Association of Naturopathic Doctors, the Canadian Association of Naturopathic Medicine, the British Columbia Association of Naturopathic Physicians, the World Society of Anti-Aging Medicine, and the International Meso-Lipotherapy Society.

Dr. Audrey Sasson, Naturopathic Doctor

Dr. Sasson provides comprehensive family practice. She completed her undergraduate degree majoring in biology and psychology and later went on to study at the Canadian College of Naturopathic Medicine in Toronto. She became licensed to practice after completing North American and Ontario licensing exams. Her practice is extensive treating patients with various concerns including: preventative medicine, diet and lifestyle modification, pain management, women's health, hormonal regulation, digestive health, immune enhancement, diabetes management and sleep disturbances.

She is an active member of the Canadian Association of Naturopathic Doctors. Dr. Sasson has completed several supplementary courses including Healthy and Active, an individualized weight loss program, and Darkfield microscopy. Dr. Sasson continues to keep current with ongoing research and clinical education attending seminars across Europe and North America.

Dr. Ana Nozari N. D.

Dr. Nozari completed her Bachelor of Science in Human Biology from the University of Toronto. She went on to receive her Doctor of Naturopathic Medicine diploma from the Canadian College of Naturopathic Medicine in 2000. She is registered to practice in Ontario and is an active member of the Ontario and Canadian Associations of Naturopathic Doctors. Her practice focus is in the areas of allergy therapy, weight loss, women's health issues, and pain management.

Christianne James, RMT., BSc., BAH., CMAG., Dip SMEP

Christianne James is the resident Integrative Manual Therapist at Pinewood Natural Health Centre.

Christianne is a licensed Canadian Osteopath and Registered Massage Therapist. She is registered with the Ontario Federation of Osteopathic Practitioners and is registered with the Canadian Massage Therapists of Ontario. She is fully certified in Contemporary Medical Acupuncture which incorporates classical acupuncture and acupuncture with electro-stimulation. As the Integrative Manual Therapist her specialties and services include: acupuncture, lymphatic drainage, cranial sacral therapy, acute and chronic pain management, trigger point therapy, myofascial release, scar therapy, cranial sacral therapy, pregnancy and pediatric massage.

Karen Gilman, Registered Holistic Nutritionist

Karen Gilman is a graduate of the Canadian School of Natural Nutrition, where she received her Diploma in Natural Nutrition. She is passionate about helping others eat well and love what they eat with an emphasis on plant-based diets, food preparation and balanced nutrition. Karen is a member of the Canadian Association of Holistic Nutrition Professionals. She is trained to assist patients with food sensitivities, digestive disorders, high cholesterol, diabetes, menopause, and inflammation.

About the Author

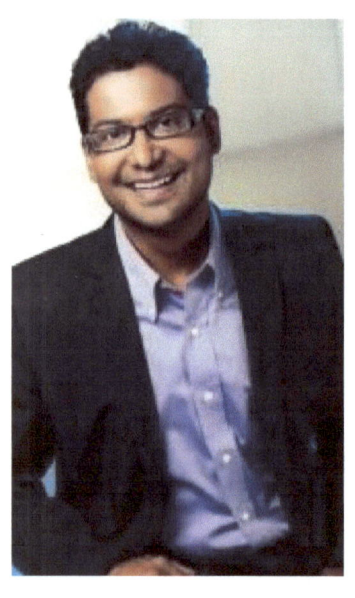

Dr. Michael Rahman, BSc, ND
Doctor of Naturopathic Medicine

Dr. Michael Rahman completed his Bachelor of Science with an emphasis on biology at McMaster University in 1993. He continued his studies at the Canadian College of Naturopathic Medicine and completed a four year doctorate program in Toronto. He is licensed to practice in both Ontario and British Columbia.

A strong interest in diagnostics and biological medicine led Dr. Rahman to further training in Biological Terrain Assessment, Darkfield Microscopy, Thermography, and advanced biological medicine and homotoxicology courses in Germany and Mexico. He then began his extensive training in mesotherapy , studying with Dr. Jacques Le Coz, MD in Paris, the direct protégé of Dr. Pistor , who originally described mesotherapy in 1952. He further studied with Dr. Patricia Rittes, MD, from Brazil, the originator of mesotherapy for fat reduction. Additional practical training from several American and South American trained physicians further developed his expertise.

Dr. Rahman founded Pinewood Natural Health Centre in

Toronto in 1997 and expanded into the Durham Region in 2003. His practice focuses on biological medicine and its treatment of chronic diseases, from fibromyalgia to cancer, and healthy age management. His practice interest also includes naturopathic cosmetic care, blending naturopathic medicine with cosmetic approaches and technology to enhance health and beauty.

Dr. Rahman is an avid lecturer and author. He lectured at the Canadian College of Naturopathic Medicine for five years: he taught microbiology to second year students and educated student clinicians in their fourth year. He has principally written technical information for other health care professionals; he has also written for local public health publications and professional journals. Dr. Rahman has also spoken at health care professional conferences throughout Canada and the United States on topics ranging from first aid to homeopathic medicine, and from fibromyalgia to cancer care.

Dr. Rahman also founded Pinewood Institute for the Advancement of Natural Therapies in 2005. He is the principal instructor teaching naturopathic doctors from across Canada and the United States mesotherapy for pain management, cosmetic mesotherapy, cosmetic Platelet Rich Plasma, and advanced homotoxicological approaches to disease.

Membership in professional organizations is important to Dr. Rahman. He is an active member of the Naturopathic Doctors Ontario, the Canadian Association of

Naturopathic Medicine, the British Columbia Association of Naturopathic Physicians, the World Society of Anti-Aging Medicine, and the International Meso-Lipotherapy Society.

References

Canadian Mental Health Association.(n.d.). [Understanding depression and its signs and symptoms]. Retrieved from: http://www.cmha.ca/mental-health/understanding-mental-illness/depression/

Canadian Sleep Society. (n.d.) [Brochures and various materials related to sleep hygiene and sleep patterns]. Retrieved from: http://www.canadiansleepsociety.ca/publisher/articlevie w/frmArticleID/341/

Canadian Society for Exercise Physiology. (n.d.).*Canadian Physical Activity Guidelines and Canadian Sedentary Behaviour Guidelines*. Retrieved from: http://www.csep.ca/english/view.asp?x=804

David, Jeanie Lerche. (2012, April 24)*Sleep Supplements: Melatonin, Valerian, and More* Retrieved from: http://www.webmd.com/vitamins-and-supplements/lifestyle-guide-11/natural-good-sleep-tips-on-melatonin-valerian

Health Canada. (2011, September 1). *Eating Well with Canada's Food Guide*. Retrieved from: http://www.hc-sc.gc.ca/fn-an/food-guide-aliment/index-eng.php

Mayo Clinic Staff. (2014, February 6). The Power of Positive Thinking. Retrieved from: http://www.mayoclinic.org/healthy-living/stress-management/in-depth/health-tip/art-20048697

What's the Difference between a Food Intolerance and Food Allergy?(2011, June 3). Retrieved from: http://www.mayoclinic.org/diseases-conditions/food-allergy/expert-answers/food-allergy/FAQ-20058538

www.ingramcontent.com/pod-product-compliance
Lightning Source LLC
Chambersburg PA
CBHW050825290526
45792CB00001B/264